SIMPLE WAY
TO
CARE FOR MYSELF

Discovering The Art Of Self-love And Holistic Well-being

By

BRAKI CRAVY

COPYRIGHT NOTICE

TABLE OF CONTENTS

INTRODUCTION

CHAPTER 1:SELF-CARE MADE EASY

CHAPTER 2:UNLOCKING THE POWER OF SELF-CARE

CHAPTER 3: NURTURING YOUR PHYSICAL HEALTH

CHAPTER 4:ENHANCING YOUR MENTAL WELL-BEING

CHAPTER 5: FUELING YOUR EMOTIONAL RESILIENCE

CHAPTER 6: PRIORITIZING SLEEP AND RELAXATION

CHAPTER 7:CULTIVATING A BALANCED LIFESTYLE

CHAPTER 8:INVESTING IN PERSONAL GROWTH

CHAPTER 9:BUILDING STRONG SUPPORT SYSTEMS

CHAPTER 10: EMBRACING MINDFULNESS AND MINDSET SHIFTS

CHAPTER 11:SELF-CARE ON THE GO (QUICK TIPS FOR BUSY INDIVIDUALS)

CHAPTER 12:CREATING SUSTAINABLE SELF-CARE HABITS

CHAPTER 13:SELF-CARE FOR EVERY SEASON

CHAPTER 14: SELF-CARE BEYOND YOURSELF

CHAPTER 15:SUSTAINING MOTIVATION AND OVERCOMING OBSTACLES

CONCLUSION

INTRODUCTION

In a quiet village set between rolling hills, there lived two remarkable friends called William and Charity. They had a special kinship and were recognized for their sensitive hearts and altruistic demeanor. Despite their philanthropic attitudes, they frequently ignored the significance of self-care.

One beautiful day, while wandering through their favorite bookshop, William happened across a book titled "Simple Way to Care for Myself." Intrigued, he couldn't resist flicking over its pages, and it was as if a whole new universe opened up before his eyes. It was a treasure mine of self-care advice and strategies.

Excited to share his unexpected finding with Charity, William immediately purchased the book and went over to Charity's home. As he retold the book's lessons, Charity's eyes expanded with every word. They were astonished to realize that taking care of oneself helped them to care for others more successfully.

Inspired and committed, William and Charity decided to go on a journey of self-care. They began gently, implementing little modifications in their everyday routines. They started each morning with a glass of cool lemon water, letting its zest revive their bodies and minds.

Embracing the power of nature, the duo regularly went for lengthy walks in the lovely countryside. The aroma of blossoming flowers and the soothing sound of chirping birds offered them a feeling of serenity and tranquility. They marveled at the beauty of their surroundings and allowed themselves to be present at the moment.

The book also stressed the need of fueling their bodies with healthy meals. William and Charity found the pleasures of making nutritious meals together, experimenting with colorful veggies, and relishing the rich tastes of fresh foods.

As they began their journey, William and Charity recognized that self-care went beyond physical concerns. They learned to carve out time for meditation and mindfulness, seeking refuge in solitude and healing their spirits.

To enhance their studies, they organized a small self-care circle with like-minded persons from their neighborhood. They shared their stories, supporting and encouraging one another along the journey. This newfound support structure helped them remain engaged and kept them responsible to prioritize their well-being.

Gradually, their lives shifted. William and Charity emanated a renewed brightness, and their good energy was captivating. People around them observed the difference and were motivated by their devotion to self-care.

Their trip not only influenced their own lives but also touched the lives of people around them. Their gestures of compassion and genuine caring grew more substantial and meaningful as they nursed themselves first. Word spread about William and Charity's change, and soon, others in the area started seeking instruction on self-care. The bookshop couldn't keep enough copies of "Simple Way to Care for Myself" in stock, as everyone wanted a piece of the magic that William and Charity had found.

Together, they arranged workshops and seminars, sharing the essential advice they had gained from the book and their own experiences. Their contagious excitement and genuine compassion pulled individuals from all walks of life, motivating them to prioritize self-care and promote kindness across the community.

The hitherto neglected notion of self-care suddenly blossomed throughout their community, producing a rippling effect of optimism and well-being. The villagers recognized that caring for themselves not only made them healthier and happier individuals but also enhanced their relationships as a community.

William and Charity's relationship became deeper as they continued to encourage and inspire one another on their self-care journey. They were glad for coming onto that tiny book, as it had initiated a metamorphosis that they never realized they needed and had immensely enhanced their lives.

And thus, the narrative of William and Charity serves as a reminder to us all that it is vital to care for ourselves to care for others wholeheartedly. With a simple book as their guide, these friends started an amazing journey of self-discovery, promoting the significance of self-care and influencing their community one act of kindness at a time. May their narrative encourage us all to prioritize our well-being and build a society where self-care and compassion go hand in hand.

puzzles, learning new abilities, or indulging in creative activities such as painting or writing. It is also crucial to emphasize mental breaks, such as practicing mindfulness or meditation, to relieve stress and increase mental clarity. Taking the time to participate in activities that provide pleasure and a feeling of success may considerably boost our mental well-being.

Caring for our emotions is sometimes forgotten yet has a critical part in our overall well-being. Acknowledging and processing our feelings is vital for sustaining mental and emotional equilibrium. This may be done by writing, talking to a trusted friend or therapist, or indulging in things that offer us pleasure and comfort. Setting appropriate boundaries and saying no to activities that deplete our emotional energy is also vital in sustaining emotional well-being.

In conclusion, applying a basic technique to care for oneself is crucial for living a satisfying and balanced life. Prioritizing physical, mental, and emotional self-care allows us to perform better in other parts of our life, such as jobs and relationships. Remembering to take pauses, participate in things that offer us pleasure, and nurture our physical and emotional well-being should not be considered a luxury, but rather a vital prerequisite for a better, happier existence.

CHAPTER 1:SELF-CARE MADE EASY

Self-care made easy is all about finding simple methods to care for myself. It doesn't have to include intricate rituals or costly therapies; it may be as basic as taking out a few minutes of the day for myself. By adding activities such as mindfulness, exercise, and prioritizing sleep, I can simply take care of myself and enhance my general well-being.

Mindfulness or meditation is a basic self-care exercise that may be done anywhere, at any time. Taking only a few minutes each day to concentrate on my breath and be present at the moment may ease tension and offer a feeling of tranquility. It enables me to become more self-aware, and I can better regulate my emotions and thoughts throughout the day.

Regular exercise is another simple method to care for myself. Engaging in physical activities like walking, running, or attending fitness courses not only helps my physical health but also raises my mood. Even a brief stroll around the block or stretching for a few minutes may make a major impact on how I feel emotionally and physically.

Indulging in modest acts of self-care throughout the day is also crucial. This may be as easy as drinking a cup of tea or coffee in the morning, relishing the flavor, and taking time for myself. Taking pauses throughout the workday to stretch, practice deep breathing, or listen to music may help replenish my mind and body, enabling me to reset and concentrate better.

One element of self-care that is frequently forgotten is prioritizing sleep. Establishing a regular sleep regimen and ensuring I receive adequate quality sleep each night is vital for my well-being. Creating a pleasant sleep environment, limiting screen time before bed, and participating in a relaxing pre-sleep ritual may all lead to improved sleep and general self-care.

It's vital to remember that self-care is not a luxury; it is a fundamental aspect of sustaining a healthy and balanced existence. By caring for myself, I am better positioned to take care of others and accomplish my tasks with clarity and passion. Making self-care a non-negotiable element of my daily routine is an investment in myself and sets a great example for others around me.

In conclusion, self-care doesn't have to be hard or time-consuming.
By combining basic practices like mindfulness, exercise, and prioritizing sleep into my everyday life, I can effortlessly care for myself. These simple actions of self-care boost not just physical and mental well-being but also increase the whole quality of my life.
So, let's make self-care a priority and experience the tremendous consequences of caring for ourselves in basic and accessible ways.

CHAPTER 2: UNLOCKING THE POWER OF SELF-CARE

In our fast-paced and demanding society, it's all too tempting to disregard our well-being. We sometimes find ourselves caught up in the rush and bustle of life, always balancing many tasks and commitments.
But among this pandemonium, it's vital to remember the significance of self-care.

Self-care involves a broad variety of activities that prioritize and nourish our physical, emotional, and mental well-being. It's about purposefully establishing time and space to refuel and refresh.
Although self-care may sometimes feel burdensome or time-consuming, there are easy methods to include it in our
everyday routines.

One such basic, but effective technique to care for oneself is the practice of mindfulness.

Mindfulness entails being completely present at the moment, paying attention to our thoughts, emotions, and body sensations without judgment. It's about anchoring ourselves in the here and now, rather than becoming buried in thoughts about the past or future.

Engaging in mindfulness may be as basic as spending a few minutes each day to sit quietly and concentrate on our breath. By noticing our breath as it goes in and out, we become more connected to our body and may ease tension and anxiety. This simple act of self-care can bring us back to our core, enabling us to reconnect with ourselves and regain a feeling of serenity and balance.

Another easy method to care for ourselves is via nourishing our physical selves. Engaging in regular exercise, even if it's only a brief stroll or light stretching, may have a dramatic influence on our general well-being. Moving our body elevates our mood, increases our energy levels, and improves our physical health. Additionally, nourishing our bodies with good meals and keeping hydrated improves our physical vigor. By prioritizing our physical health, we are actively investing in our long-term well-being.

Taking time for things that offer us joy and pleasure is also a crucial element of self-care. Engaging in hobbies, such as painting, cooking, or playing an instrument, helps us to tap into our creative side and gives us an opportunity for self-expression. These hobbies create a feeling of satisfaction and give us a much-needed reprieve from the stresses of everyday life.

Finally, it's vital to appreciate the value of establishing boundaries and saying no when required. Taking on too many obligations or continually compromising our own needs may lead to exhaustion and discontent. By being forceful and prioritizing our own needs, we are playing an active part in our self-care journey.

In conclusion, unlocking the potential of self-care starts with implementing basic routines into our everyday lives. By practicing mindfulness, nourishing our physical bodies, participating in things that please us, and establishing boundaries, we may successfully care for ourselves and enjoy the advantages of enhanced well-being. Remember, self-care is not selfish, but rather a critical investment in ourselves that eventually helps us to show up fully for others and lead a more fulfilling life.

CHAPTER 3: NURTURING YOUR PHYSICAL HEALTH

Nurturing your physical health is a critical component of caring for yourself, and happily, there are easy methods to do it. Taking care of your physical health not only enhances your general well-being but also energizes you and helps you to fully participate in your everyday activities.

One easy strategy to nourish your physical health is by prioritizing regular exercise. Engaging in physical exercise not only helps you maintain a healthy weight but also improves your cardiovascular health, strength, and flexibility. You don't have to spend hours at the gym or engage in high-intensity exercises to gain the advantages of exercise. Simple exercises like walking, running, or cycling for at least 30 minutes a day may dramatically enhance your physical well-being. Find an exercise regimen that complements your lifestyle and hobbies, and you'll be more likely to continue with it.

Another straightforward strategy to care for yourself physically is by choosing a balanced and healthy diet. Fueling your body with entire meals, such as fruits, vegetables, lean proteins, whole grains, and healthy fats, supplies it with the required nutrients to perform efficiently. Avoid or restrict your consumption of processed meals, sugary snacks, and drinks rich in added sugars, since they may lead to weight gain and different health risks. Additionally, remain hydrated by consuming a proper quantity of water throughout the day.

In addition to exercise and a balanced diet, obtaining adequate sleep is vital for maintaining your physical health. Aim for a regular sleep routine and attempt to obtain roughly 7-8 hours of quality sleep each night. A good night's sleep rejuvenates your body, boosts cognitive performance, and helps manage your emotions. Establishing a nocturnal routine, having a peaceful and pleasant sleep environment, and avoiding technology before bed may lead to improved sleep quality.

Furthermore, regulating stress is vital for your physical wellness.
Chronic stress may lead to different health concerns, including cardiovascular troubles, reduced immune systems, and sleep disorders. Implementing stress-reducing practices, such as meditation, deep breathing exercises, spending time in nature, or indulging in hobbies, may dramatically enhance your general well-being. It's crucial to take pauses, prioritize self-care, and find appropriate outlets for stress management.

Lastly, do not underestimate the need for frequent check-ups and preventive screenings. Visiting your healthcare practitioner regularly enables early diagnosis and prevention of any health conditions. It is also a fantastic time to share any concerns or questions you may have regarding your physical health.

Nurturing your physical health via basic self-care routines is an investment in your entire well-being and quality of life. By emphasizing regular exercise, adopting a balanced diet, getting enough sleep, controlling stress, and obtaining regular medical treatment, you may take proactive efforts towards nurturing your physical health.

Remember, even tiny adjustments may make a significant impact, so start adopting these basic practices into your daily routine and watch as your physical health and energy grow.

In conclusion, supporting your physical health is a key component of caring for yourself.
By combining basic habits such as regular exercise, balanced diet, adequate sleep, stress management, and regular check-ups, you may efficiently care for your physical well-being.

Remember, taking little measures towards a healthy lifestyle may lead to major changes in your overall health and vigor. Prioritize your physical health and watch as you flourish and experience a greater quality of life.

CHAPTER 4:ENHANCING YOUR MENTAL WELL-BEING

Enhancing your mental well-being is a crucial component of caring for oneself. In today's fast-paced and demanding society, it is vital to prioritize your mental health as much as your physical health. Simple activities and habits may greatly help to increase your mental well-being and general pleasure.

Firstly, exercising self-care is an excellent strategy to boost your mental well-being. Allocating time each day for things that you love and calm you, such as reading a book, having a long bath, or practicing meditation, may help decrease stress and enhance your mood.

Taking care of your physical health, like getting enough sleep, eating healthy meals, and exercising frequently, is also a vital element of self-care since it directly affects your mental well-being.

Furthermore, engaging with people is another easy but effective technique to increase your mental well-being.

Building and sustaining good connections may give you a feeling of belonging and support, which are vital for your mental health. Reach out to loved ones often, spend quality time with them, and participate in activities that foster social contact. This might entail joining a club or community organization, engaging in team sports, or just having a coffee meeting with a buddy.

Additionally, finding appropriate strategies to handle stress is crucial for your mental well-being. Stress may take a toll on your mental health, leading to anxiety, depression, and other disorders. Engaging in activities that help you relax and unwind, such as practicing mindfulness methods, deep breathing exercises, or engaging in a pastime you like, may help lower stress levels and produce a feeling of peace.

Setting realistic objectives and concentrating on personal progress is another component of increasing your mental well-being. By defining reasonable objectives and working towards them, you may develop a feeling of purpose and success, which can favorably improve your self-esteem and general mental health. Whether it's learning a new skill, following a hobby, or improving your work, having objectives may give direction and inspiration in your life.

Lastly, it's crucial to take pauses and allow yourself time to refuel. In our fast-paced environment, it's easy to get overwhelmed and burned out. Taking pauses helps you to relax and revitalize, leading to better productivity and a clearer mentality. Whether it's taking a stroll in nature, practicing relaxation methods, or just finding a peaceful area to sit in solitude, giving yourself frequent breaks may be a simple but powerful approach to care for your mental well-being.

Finally, boosting your mental well-being is a key aspect of caring for yourself. By practicing self-care, interacting with people, managing stress, creating goals, and taking breaks, you may develop a healthy attitude and overall happiness. Remember, taking modest efforts to care for yourself psychologically may have a tremendous influence on your well-being. Prioritize your mental health, and you'll find yourself more able to tackle the stresses of life and enjoy a greater quality of life.

CHAPTER 5: FUELING YOUR EMOTIONAL RESILIENCE

In our hurried and frequently disorganized environment, it is easy to disregard our mental health. As we navigate through daily problems, it becomes vital to prioritize self-care.

Fueling emotional resilience is a key element of our self-care regimen, helping us to bounce back from setbacks and confront hardship with power and grace. As I endeavor to care for myself, I have found a simple but efficient technique to develop and preserve my emotional resilience.

The first step in feeding my emotional resilience is identifying and embracing my feelings. I have learned that concealing or rejecting what I feel simply leads to emotional tiredness and more major difficulties down the line. Instead, I welcome all my feelings, whether joyful or bad, as useful and helpful. By allowing myself to feel, I may understand myself better and find the fundamental reasons for my feelings. This self-awareness helps me to react to situations more effectively, as I gain insight into my triggers and create healthy coping techniques.

Another key part of feeding my emotional resilience is establishing a support network. It is vital to surround oneself with persons that elevate and encourage me on my quest. These folks might be friends, family members, or even professional mentors who give direction and encouragement.

Sharing my experiences and feelings with these trustworthy persons helps me to obtain various views and insights, enabling me to navigate through challenging circumstances with enhanced resilience. Additionally, having a strong support network creates a feeling of belonging and community, which is vital for sustaining mental well-being.

Practicing self-care routines is also a critical element of feeding my emotional resiliency. Taking time for myself and indulging in things that offer me pleasure and relaxation is a wonderful method to refill my emotional supplies. Whether it is reading a book, going on a stroll in nature, doing yoga, or indulging in a pastime, these times of self-care help me refuel and develop emotional strength. Regularly participating in these activities guarantees that I can confront problems with a clear head and a good outlook.

Furthermore, developing a development attitude is crucial in fuelling my emotional resilience. Adopting a perspective that obstacles are opportunities for development and learning encourages me to tackle failures with perseverance and resolve. Instead of perceiving setbacks as personal faults, I see them as stepping stones toward personal and emotional growth.

By reframing my mentality, I am more able to bounce back from adversity and discover solutions to issues, rather than concentrating on the bad elements.

Lastly, cultivating thankfulness is a wonderful method to feed emotional resilience. Taking time each day to think about and express appreciation for the things I value in life helps change my perspective from negative to positive. This simple exercise helps me retain perspective and reminds me of the wealth in my life, especially during hard times. Instead of obsessing over what went wrong, I refocus my attention on what I am thankful for, developing a feeling of emotional resilience and hope.

Fueling my emotional resilience is a continual and conscious activity.
As I prioritize my emotional well-being, I am better ready to negotiate life's inevitable ups and downs with strength and grace. By noticing and embracing my feelings, building a support network, practicing self-care, maintaining a growth mindset, and expressing appreciation, I am continually fuelling my emotional resilience and assuring a better, happier me.

This simple technique of caring for myself not only helps me but also enables me to show up as the greatest version of myself in my relationships and contribute positively to the world around me.

CHAPTER 6: PRIORITIZING SLEEP AND RELAXATION

Prioritizing sleep and relaxation is an important element of self-care. In this day and age, it is easy to overlook the necessity of obtaining proper relaxation. However, making sleep and relaxation a priority in your daily routine may have several advantages for your general well-being.

Getting adequate sleep is vital for our bodies and brains to operate efficiently. It is during sleep that our bodies mend themselves, refresh energy levels, and solidify memories.

Lack of sleep may lead to lower productivity, poor cognitive function, emotional swings, a damaged immune system, and a higher risk of accidents. By prioritizing sleep, you are providing your body the essential time to repair and revitalize, which eventually increases your physical and mental performance.

Besides getting adequate sleep, including relaxation into your routine is crucial.

In today's hectic society, stress has become a daily occurrence. Chronic stress may take a toll on both your physical and emotional health. Engaging in relaxation exercises helps to combat the detrimental impacts of stress. It provides your body an opportunity to relax and heal, resulting in less muscular tension, lower blood pressure, increased immunological function, and enhanced mood.

There are various easy strategies to prioritize sleep and relaxation in your everyday life. Firstly, maintain a regular sleep routine by going to bed and getting up at the same time every day, including weekends. This helps adjust your body's internal clock and promotes greater sleep quality.

Secondly, build a calming nighttime ritual that informs your body it's time to unwind and prepare for sleep. This may include things such as reading a book, having a warm bath, practicing meditation or deep breathing techniques, or listening to relaxing music. Avoid devices and stimulating activities close to bedtime, since they might interfere with your sleep.

Additionally, make your sleep environment favorable to slumber. Ensure your bedroom is cold, dark, and quiet. Use comfy pillows and a sturdy mattress. Limit noise and light interruptions, and consider using blackout curtains, earplugs, or white noise devices if required.

Incorporating relaxation methods into your routine may help boost general well-being. Find things that help you relax and destress, such as practicing yoga, indulging in regular physical exercise, going for walks in nature, or spending time on hobbies that you like. Prioritize time for self-care activities and make them non-negotiable in your calendar.

Lastly, avoid overcommitting yourself and learn to say no when necessary. Overloading your schedule may lead to elevated stress levels and restricted time for relaxation. Prioritizing sleep and relaxation means establishing boundaries and making self-care a priority.

In conclusion, prioritizing sleep and relaxation is a simple but effective method to care for oneself. It not only promotes your physical and mental well-being but also boosts your overall productivity and happiness. By making sleep a priority, practicing relaxation methods, and including self-care activities in your routine, you may enjoy the numerous advantages that come with taking care of yourself. Remember, rest is not luxuries but a need for a healthy and balanced existence.

CHAPTER 7:CULTIVATING A BALANCED LIFESTYLE

Cultivating a balanced lifestyle is vital for general well-being and enjoyment. It entails preserving harmony between diverse parts of life, such as jobs, relationships, personal hobbies, and physical and mental health. In the middle of our hectic lives, it is easy to feel overwhelmed and overlook our own needs. However, by following a basic technique to care for ourselves, we may build a balanced lifestyle and enjoy a more happy existence.

The first step in building a healthy lifestyle is to prioritize self-care. This requires identifying and addressing our own needs and making them a priority. It might be as easy as allocating a few minutes each day to indulge in things that offer us pleasure and calm. This might be reading a book, going on a stroll outside, practicing meditation or yoga, or enjoying a hobby. Prioritizing self-care guarantees that we are investing in our well-being, which eventually helps us to better care for others and accomplish our duties.

Another crucial part of having a balanced lifestyle is establishing appropriate limits. This includes learning to say no when required and recognizing our limitations. It is vital to create boundaries in relationships, in work, and in other aspects of life to avoid burnout and maintain a healthy balance. By being firm and stating our requirements, we may prevent over-committing ourselves and enduring unneeded stress.

In addition, establishing a balance between job and personal life is crucial for a well-rounded life. This includes defining clear boundaries between the two and allocating attention to both areas. It involves avoiding overworking or carrying work-related stress home, as well as ensuring that personal time is restorative and pleasurable. By separating work and personal life, we may develop a more harmonic balance that helps us to succeed in all aspects of life.

Physical health is also a vital aspect of a balanced lifestyle. Engaging in regular exercise, eating a good diet, and getting adequate sleep are necessary for overall physical well-being. Making time for physical exercise, even if it is a brief walk or stretching session, may enhance energy levels, improve mood, and lessen the risk of numerous health conditions.

Nourishing the body with good meals and prioritizing appropriate sleep guarantees that we have the energy and vigor to explore all facets of life.

Lastly, emotional and mental well-being are vital components of a balanced lifestyle. Taking care of our mental health entails learning to handle stress, practicing self-compassion, and getting assistance when required. Engaging in things that offer us pleasure, such as spending time with loved ones, pursuing hobbies, and practicing mindfulness or journaling, may also contribute to emotional well-being. Additionally, developing strong connections and surrounding oneself with a supportive network of friends and family may tremendously benefit our mental health.

In all, creating a balanced lifestyle is a simple approach to caring for ourselves.
By emphasizing self-care, creating boundaries, balancing work and personal life, concentrating on physical health, and fostering emotional well-being, we may build a life that is harmonious, rewarding, and sustainable.

Remember, it is not about attaining perfection in every element, but rather striking a healthy balance that enables us to flourish and appreciate everything that life has to offer.

CHAPTER 8:INVESTING IN PERSONAL GROWTH

Investing in personal improvement is a simple but significant method to care for oneself. Just as we fuel our bodies with nutritious food and exercise, it is equally crucial to prioritize our mental, emotional, and spiritual well-being. By making a deliberate effort to engage in personal development, we are enabling ourselves to expand, learn, and prosper in all parts of life.

One of the easiest ways to care for ourselves is to commit to lifelong learning. Education does not stop with a degree or certification; it is a constant journey that develops our thoughts and widens our perspectives. Whether it be reading books, attending seminars, or enrolling in online courses, devoting time and effort to obtaining new information may lead to personal growth and development.

Another crucial part of human development is self-reflection. Taking the time to introspect and understand oneself is vital for emotional intelligence and self-awareness. Engaging in activities such as meditation, writing, or seeking counseling may bring useful insights into our thoughts, feelings, and patterns of behavior. By having a greater awareness of ourselves, we may make intentional decisions that match our beliefs and ambitions.

Furthermore, investing in personal improvement includes surrounding oneself with good influences. The company we keep tremendously impacts our attitudes, beliefs, and behaviors. Building a supporting network of friends, mentors, or like-minded persons may bring encouragement, inspiration, and a feeling of belonging. Engaging in meaningful discussions, seeking direction, and exchanging experiences with people who are likewise committed to personal progress may substantially benefit our path.

Additionally, pushing oneself is a vital aspect of personal development.

Stepping out of our comfort zones and accepting new experiences helps us to grow our abilities, knowledge, and views. Whether it's taking up a new activity, attempting a fresh approach to problem-solving, or taking on a project that challenges our limitations, pushing ourselves beyond what we believed possible may lead to enormous personal development.

Investing in personal development also entails taking care of our physical well-being. As the adage goes, "A healthy mind dwells in a healthy body." Engaging in regular exercise, prioritizing sleep, and practicing self-care activities like good eating and relaxation methods may greatly improve our overall well-being.

When we feel physically strong and energetic, it becomes simpler to concentrate on personal progress and welcome new challenges.

In conclusion, investing in personal development is a simple but crucial method to care for ourselves. By valuing lifelong learning, self-reflection, good relationships, difficult experiences, and physical well-being, we may support personal growth and development. This not only benefits our personal lives but also helps us to show up as our best selves in our relationships, professions, and all aspects of life. So, let us commit to investing in personal improvement as a method to care for ourselves and nourish our growth and well-being.

CHAPTER 9:BUILDING STRONG SUPPORT SYSTEMS

Building solid support networks is a vital component when it comes to caring for oneself. Taking care of oneself entails more than simply physical well-being; it also includes nourishing one's emotional, mental, and social qualities. And having a solid support system may give the essential basis to guarantee all these demands are addressed.

The first step in building a healthy support system is identifying the persons who uplift and encourage us. These folks might be family members, friends, or even mentors who cheer us on and lend a listening ear when required. Surrounding oneself with good and helpful folks may considerably contribute to our general well-being.

Additionally, it's crucial to explain our requirements to individuals inside our support system. Whether it's expressing our feelings, seeking guidance, or just asking for assistance, opening up and being vulnerable with people helps develop better ties. Clear and honest communication helps people to understand our needs and give the assistance we seek.

Another crucial part of having a good support system is diversifying it. Relying on just one or two individuals for assistance may be problematic, since their capacity to be there for us may be restricted owing to their duties and commitments. By building connections with numerous persons, we enhance the odds of having someone accessible when we need them most.

Furthermore, it is crucial to note that support networks may extend beyond only individuals. Engaging in activities or hobbies that offer pleasure and satisfaction may operate as a support system in itself. Taking the time to care for oneself via self-care techniques such as exercise, meditation, or creative outlets may be extremely useful for mental and emotional well-being.

Lastly, being a member of a community or support group may be essential in developing a solid support system. These communities give a feeling of belonging, understanding, and shared experiences, which may greatly help one's self-care journey. Options for joining such groups may be found through local organizations, internet platforms, or seeking expert help.

Developing strong support networks is a simple but vital method to care for oneself. It entails recognizing supportive persons, developing open communication, diversifying support networks, participating in self-care activities, and being a part of supportive communities.
By purposefully investing in these connections and resources, we may guarantee our overall well-being is cultivated and maintained.

CHAPTER 10: EMBRACING MINDFULNESS AND MINDSET SHIFTS

In our fast-paced society packed with continual demands and diversions, it's easy to get caught up in the turmoil and forget to take care of ourselves. However, one easy yet effective method to care for ourselves is through adopting mindfulness and making mental modifications.

Mindfulness refers to the discipline of being completely present and aware of our thoughts, emotions, and experiences in the present moment, without judgment. It entails paying attention to our thoughts and feelings and accepting them as they are, without attempting to alter or control them. When we are aware, we can build a feeling of serenity and clarity, and we become more responsive to our wants and desires.

So how can we embrace mindfulness? There are several methods to bring mindfulness into our everyday life. One helpful strategy is to participate in meditation or deep breathing exercises.

Allocating only a few minutes each day to sit quietly and concentrate on our breath may help us become more focused and grounded. Additionally, practicing mindfulness during ordinary tasks such as eating, walking, or even cleaning dishes may offer a feeling of presence and gratitude for these basic moments.

Alongside mindfulness, thinking modifications play a significant part in caring for oneself. Our mentality is the lens through which we observe and interpret the world. By adopting a positive mentality, we may improve our view and boost our general well-being.

One beneficial thinking adjustment is practicing appreciation. Taking a few minutes each day to concentrate on what we are thankful for might transform our perspective and remind us of the numerous benefits in our life. It may help us concentrate on the good qualities and promote a feeling of satisfaction.

Another mentality adjustment is practicing self-compassion. Often, we are our own toughest critics, continually evaluating ourselves and berating ourselves for perceived defects or failures. However, fostering an attitude of self-compassion entails treating oneself with love and empathy, just as we would a good friend. It involves accepting our shortcomings and errors without judgment and providing ourselves with forgiveness and support.

Furthermore, having a development attitude may be very advantageous. This mentality entails faith in our potential to learn, develop, and improve. Rather than perceiving problems or setbacks as failures, we embrace them as opportunities for growth and development.
By moving our emphasis from results to the process of learning and personal development,

we may create a feeling of resilience and optimism.By adopting mindfulness and making mental modifications, we may build a simple but effective strategy to care for ourselves. These techniques assist us to slow down, listen in, and prioritize our well-being amid life's pressures.

In conclusion, caring for oneself is not necessarily about lavish self-indulgence or elaborate procedures. By adopting mindfulness and making mental modifications, we may build a simple but powerful approach to caring for ourselves.

Practicing mindfulness allows us to be present in the moment, build tranquility, and better comprehend our thoughts and emotions. It might be as easy as spending a few seconds each day to concentrate on our breath or being completely involved in regular tasks.

CHAPTER 11:SELF-CARE ON THE GO (QUICK TIPS FOR BUSY INDIVIDUALS)

Maintaining self-care is crucial, especially for busy people. While it may seem tough to make time for oneself with a crowded schedule, there are easy methods to care for yourself on the move.

Here are some brief recommendations for busy adults wishing to prioritize self-care:

Start Your Day With Intention

Begin each day by making good objectives. Take a few minutes in the morning to think about the day ahead and imagine a successful and rewarding day. This exercise may help create a pleasant tone and mentality for the day.

Practice Awareness

Incorporate moments of mindfulness throughout your day. Instead of hurrying from one work to another, spend a few minutes to completely participate in the present moment. Pay attention to your environment, your senses, and your thoughts. This technique may help relieve stress and boost your general well-being.

Take Tiny Breaks

Schedule brief breaks throughout the day. These pauses might be as brief as five minutes. Use this time to move away from work, stretch or take a brief stroll, and clear your head. These mini-breaks may enhance productivity and energy levels.

Embrace Self-compassion

Be gentle and empathetic towards oneself. Understand that you are doing the best you can with the time and resources available to you. Treat yourself with the same tenderness and compassion you would show to a loved one. Remind yourself that it's appropriate to take pauses and prioritize self-care.

Find Moments Of Delight

Seek moments of joy and pleasure throughout your day. It may be as easy as drinking a wonderful cup of coffee, listening to your favorite music during your commute, or spending a few minutes indulging in a hobby or activity you like. These moments of delight might help increase your mood and general well-being.

Practice Self-care Rituals

Incorporate little self-care routines into your everyday routine. It may be anything as easy as applying a scented lotion, spending a few minutes to stretch or perform some moderate yoga postures, or having a warm bath or shower. These routines may bring a sensation of calm and regeneration.

Delegate And Seek Help

Recognize that you don't have to accomplish it all by yourself. Delegate chores wherever feasible, whether it's at work or home. Ask for aid when you need it. By sharing duties and finding help, you may free up crucial time for self-care.

Prioritize What Matters Most

Take a step back and analyze your priorities. Determine what is important to you and align your actions and choices appropriately. Eliminate unneeded commitments and responsibilities that don't correspond with your ideals or offer you pleasure. By prioritizing what is genuinely important, you may make more space and time for self-care.

Remember, self-care doesn't have to be complex or time-consuming. It's about finding little moments to prioritize your well-being and recharge, even in the middle of a hectic schedule. By applying these easy steps, you can care for yourself on the road and maintain a healthy and balanced lifestyle.

CHAPTER 12:CREATING SUSTAINABLE SELF-CARE HABITS

Creating lasting self-care practices is a simple but vital approach to caring for oneself. In today's fast-paced and demanding environment, it's easy to feel overwhelmed and overlook our well-being. However, taking the time to build sustainable self-care habits is vital for boosting physical, mental, and emotional wellness.

One of the first stages in building lasting self-care routines is to prioritize your needs. It's crucial to know that self-care is not a luxury but a need. We typically put the demands of others or our job above our well-being, which ultimately leads to burnout and exhaustion. By realizing that self-care should be a priority, we may start making intentional efforts to care for ourselves regularly and sustainably.

Identify hobbies that offer you pleasure and relaxation. The beauty of self-care is that it may vary for everyone. Some folks find consolation in hobbies such as yoga, meditation, or reading, while others may prefer going for a run, making a nutritious meal, or practicing a hobby. Experiment with various hobbies to find what resonates with you and meets your requirements. It's vital to find activities that are sustainable and readily fit into your daily schedule.

Establishing a routine is another key part of building lasting self-care behaviors. Consistency is crucial in making self-care a sustainable practice. Decide on particular periods of the day or week that are devoted completely to self-care. Whether it's setting aside 30 minutes every morning for meditation or booking an hour each Sunday for a lengthy walk in nature, establishing a schedule helps to embed these self-care activities in your regular life.

It's also crucial to be realistic and adaptable while building lasting self-care practices. Life may be unpredictable, and there will be instances when your routine is upset or unforeseen obstacles occur. Rather than fully abandoning your self-care regimen in these instances, be open to altering it to match your present circumstances. This might mean choosing shorter but still rewarding hobbies, changing your routine to meet a new time of day, or including self-care routines that can be easily done on the go.

Additionally, it's vital to realize that self-care extends beyond simply physical activity. Nurturing your mental and emotional well-being is equally crucial.

This might entail practicing positive affirmations, getting treatment or counseling when required, building healthy relationships, and setting boundaries with others. Prioritizing time for self-reflection and introspection may also help to lasting self-care practices, as it enables you to frequently review your needs and make modifications as required.

Lastly, check that your self-care behaviors correspond with your beliefs and ambitions. Take the time to focus on what is important to you and what you desire to accomplish in life. By combining self-care activities that connect with your beliefs and support your objectives, you are more likely to remain motivated and dedicated to doing them regularly.

Creating sustained self-care practices is not about indulging in occasional indulgences or short-term remedies.
It is about committing to care for oneself in a comprehensive and long-lasting approach. By prioritizing your needs, identifying activities that bring you joy and relaxation, establishing a routine, being realistic and flexible, nurturing your mental and emotional well-being, and aligning your self-care habits with your values, you can create sustainable self-care habits that will contribute to your overall well-being and happiness.
Remember, caring for oneself is not selfish but vital for living a full and balanced life.

CHAPTER 13:SELF-CARE FOR EVERY SEASON

Change is an unavoidable aspect of life, and with each season comes new difficulties and possibilities.

As human beings, we must learn to adapt to these changes to flourish and retain our well-being. One of the most effective ways to negotiate these transitions is by practicing self-care. Taking care of oneself is not a luxury but a need, and by applying basic self-care routines, we can adjust to each season of life with ease.

Self-care is not about engaging in costly hobbies or spending hours on end pampering ourselves. It is about actively choosing decisions that promote our physical, emotional, and mental well. In every season of life, new parts of self-care become more apparent, and it is vital to alter our habits accordingly.

In the spring, a season of fresh beginnings and development, self-care may concentrate on rebirth and revitalization. Taking a stroll in nature, practicing yoga or meditation, and feeding our bodies with fresh, seasonal foods are all easy but effective methods to care for ourselves at this time. The idea is to check in to our body and pay attention to what we need to feel invigorated and renewed.

As summer arrives, a season of warmth and plenty, self-care might turn towards relaxing and appreciating the simple joys in life. Taking a day off to go to the beach, reading a book outside, or spending time with loved ones may all add to a feeling of well-being and regeneration during this season. It is crucial to emphasize relaxation and leisure activities, enabling oneself to recuperate and completely appreciate the delights of summer.

In the fall, a season of transition and transformation, self-care might concentrate on meditation and introspection.

Taking the time to write, practice gratitude, or participate in creative activities may help us process our feelings and negotiate any shifts that may come our way. It is also crucial to adopt healthy habits and rituals throughout this season, such as regular exercise, good sleep, and nutritional meals, to offer a feeling of stability and support during times of transition.

Finally, when winter approaches, a season of silence and contemplation, self-care may revolve around nurturing and self-compassion. indulging in activities that provide comfort and warmth, such as taking long baths, practicing mindfulness, or indulging in hobbies that bring delight, may help us traverse the colder, darker months with grace and self-care.
Supporting our immune systems via healthy eating and being active may also play a crucial part in self-care throughout the winter season.

Adapting to change demands flexibility and a willingness to prioritize our well-being. By implementing basic self-care techniques into our daily routines, we may better adjust to the ever-changing seasons of life. It is crucial to remember that self-care is not a one-size-fits-all idea; what works for one person may not work for another. Therefore, it is crucial to listen to our own needs and alter our self-care habits appropriately.

It is not selfish to practice self-care, but rather an act of self-protection. By taking care of ourselves, we are better prepared to show up for others and face the obstacles that come with change. So, whether it's a simple act of self-care like taking a 10-minute stroll, engaging in a beloved activity, or just taking a few deep breaths, let's prioritize our well-being and adapt to each season with grace and self-love.

CHAPTER 14: SELF-CARE BEYOND YOURSELF

In popular culture, self-care is typically connected with indulging in pleasures or pampering oneself. While this is vital to refresh and recharge, self-care should also extend beyond ourselves to include contributing to the community we live in. By actively engaging in our community and assisting others, we not only boost our well-being but also generate a beneficial influence on the world around us.

One easy method to care for ourselves while giving to society is by performing small acts of kindness. These gestures might range from lending a listening ear to a buddy in need, volunteering at a local charity, or helping someone with their shopping. Such tiny acts may have a huge influence on someone's day and build a feeling of connectedness and empathy in our society. It is a win-win scenario, as we not only provide enjoyment to others but also feel a sense of satisfaction and purpose inside ourselves.

Engaging in community service is another wonderful method to care for ourselves while giving back. By giving time and effort to organizations or issues that correspond with our beliefs, we receive a feeling of purpose and make a meaningful impact in the lives of others. Whether it is educating youngsters, cleaning up the environment, or offering support to the elderly, there are endless ways to contribute to the welfare of our community.

By donating our talents and resources to people in need, we not only enhance the lives of others but also raise our own self-esteem and personal development.

Supporting local businesses is another easy but powerful method to care for ourselves and contribute to the community. By choosing to buy at small businesses and institutions instead of giant companies, we help promote the local economy and build a flourishing community.

Local companies frequently provide distinctive goods and services that represent the culture and values of the community, generating a feeling of identification and pride. Moreover, by supporting local businesses, we help to job development and economic sustainability in our region.

Lastly, exercising self-care outside ourselves includes pushing for good change and addressing societal challenges. By increasing awareness about vital problems such as mental health, equality, or environmental protection, we become catalysts for change within our community. Whether it is by sharing information on social media, joining protests, or engaging in meaningful discussions, we can impact and inspire others. By educating ourselves and others, we foster empathy, understanding, and a feeling of social responsibility.

In conclusion, self-care should not be restricted to our preferences and requirements. By extending our care and concern to our community, we not only boost our well-being but also generate a beneficial influence on the world around us. Simple acts of kindness, participating in community service, supporting local businesses, and pushing for social change are all ways in which we may contribute to the good of our community while caring for ourselves. By doing so, we establish a circle of compassion, connection, and development that benefits not just ourselves but also the collective well-being of our community.

CHAPTER 15:SUSTAINING MOTIVATION AND OVERCOMING OBSTACLES

Sustaining motivation and overcoming hurdles are essential components when it comes to caring for oneself. In the quest for self-care, it is typical to confront hurdles that may hamper our progress or diminish our excitement.
However, by learning how to preserve motivation and overcome these difficulties, we may guarantee that the basic approach to care for ourselves stays a continuous and pleasant habit.

One of the major keys to retaining motivation is to create realistic and attainable objectives. When making objectives for self-care, it is crucial to find hobbies or practices that connect with us individually. It might be as easy as going for a walk every day, performing deep breathing techniques, or committing time to indulge in an activity we like.

By matching our objectives with our interests and passions, we are more likely to remain motivated and involved in our self-care practice.

Additionally, it is crucial to recognize tiny accomplishments along the road. Acknowledging and thanking ourselves for reaching even the smallest goals may dramatically enhance our drive. By doing so, we produce positive reinforcement and establish a feeling of pride in our self-care journey. This attitude may inspire our enthusiasm and drive to continue caring for ourselves in a basic but significant way.

However, despite our best efforts, difficulties may develop that test our desire and readiness to exercise self-care. These hurdles might vary from external considerations such as time limits, professional obligations, or family duties, to internal barriers such as self-doubt or lack of confidence. Regardless of the nature of these difficulties, it is crucial to have solutions in place to overcome them.

One effective technique to overcome problems is to establish a positive mentality. Remind yourself of the advantages of self-care and the beneficial influence it has on your overall well-being. By concentrating on the positive elements, you may transform your attitude from seeing difficulties as problems to perceiving them as chances for development and self-improvement.

Another method is to seek help from others. Reach out to friends, family, or a support network who can give insight, encouragement, and accountability. Sharing your self-care journey with others not only creates a feeling of community but also provides an outlet for obtaining helpful advice or insights from those who may have conquered similar hurdles in their own life.

Furthermore, it is crucial to be flexible and adaptive in your self-care regimen. Life is full of unexpected twists and turns, and it is vital to alter your self-care habits to meet your present circumstances. This may require finding innovative methods to integrate self-care activities into your daily routine, or altering your objectives to make them more attainable and practical. By being adaptable, you can guarantee that self-care remains a priority even in the face of hurdles.

Lastly, practicing self-compassion is vital while negotiating challenges in the self-care path. Understand that failures and struggles are a normal part of life, and it is alright to stumble along the road. Instead of blaming yourself or giving up, offer yourself care and empathy. Treat yourself with the same kindness and assistance you would provide a friend experiencing comparable problems.
By practicing self-compassion, you may bounce back from failures and continue caring for yourself with fresh drive and resilience.

In conclusion, retaining motivation and overcoming barriers are key components of a simple approach to caring for oneself. By establishing realistic objectives, appreciating little accomplishments, maintaining a positive mentality, seeking assistance, being adaptable, and practicing self-compassion, we may overcome any hurdles that emerge on our self-care path. With persistence and resilience, we can guarantee that caring for ourselves stays a priority, leading to better well-being and a happier, more full existence.

CONCLUSION

Throughout this articles, we have studied the several easy ways we may care for ourselves and go on the road to becoming happier and healthier humans. From physical self-care routines to supporting our mental and emotional well-being, each action we take adds to our total well-being.

Self-care is a comprehensive notion that involves both our physical and mental wellness. Taking care of our bodies entails fundamental behaviors such as getting adequate sleep, eating good meals, and participating in regular exercise. These small behaviors may have a major influence on our energy levels, emotions, and general health. By prioritizing these parts of our life, we develop a firm foundation for a happier and healthier self.

Equally vital is the care we offer to our mental and emotional well-being. Stress management practices including practicing mindfulness, participating in activities we like, and getting help from loved ones or specialists are vital to our mental health. Prioritizing self-care in this area assists us to build resilience and better dealing with life's obstacles.

It is crucial to remember that self-care is neither selfish nor indulgent; rather, it is a critical investment in ourselves. By making ourselves a priority, we are more able to serve and care for those in our life. In our fast-paced and demanding environment, it is tempting to disregard our own needs and emphasize the needs of others. However, we must know that we cannot pour from an empty cup. Taking the effort to care for ourselves helps us to show up as our best selves for our loved ones and the world around us.

Implementing self-care techniques may not always be simple, particularly if we are used to putting others before ourselves. It involves a change in perspective and a commitment to make yourself a priority. However, the benefits are worth it. By taking care of ourselves, we not only enjoy greater physical health, but also build a feeling of contentment, inner calm, and pleasure.

Self-care is an ongoing endeavor that requires consistent effort and wise choices. It is not something that can be done just once and forgotten. It is crucial to be gentle with ourselves and remember that self-care looks different for everyone. What works for one person may not work for another, thus it is vital to research and find what methods connect with us.

As we complete our investigation of self-care and its role in our path toward a happier and healthier self, it is vital to reflect on the progress we have made and the changes we have undertaken. Celebrate even the slightest achievements, because they are building blocks on our journey to personal progress.

Remember that self-care is not a destination but a continuous practice.

It is a continuing path of self-discovery, self-compassion, and self-improvement.
Each day gives us a chance to prioritize ourselves and make decisions that accord with our well-being.

Your road to a happy, healthier self starts with simple actions and habits. By adopting physical self-care routines, nourishing your mental and emotional well-being, and making yourself a priority, you are taking big advances towards a more satisfying existence.
Embrace this adventure with an open mind and a compassionate heart. Be nice to yourself, be patient with yourself, and celebrate your success along the road.

It is essential to recognize that self-care is not a mere indulgence, but a necessity. You deserve to live a life that is joyful, healthy, and by your actual self.

So, go on this road with confidence, dedication, and a commitment to yourself. Embrace the simplicity of self-care and watch as it affects your life for the better. You are capable of obtaining pleasure and health, and you deserve every bit of it.